Paleo Diet

I0450535

Old is Gold!

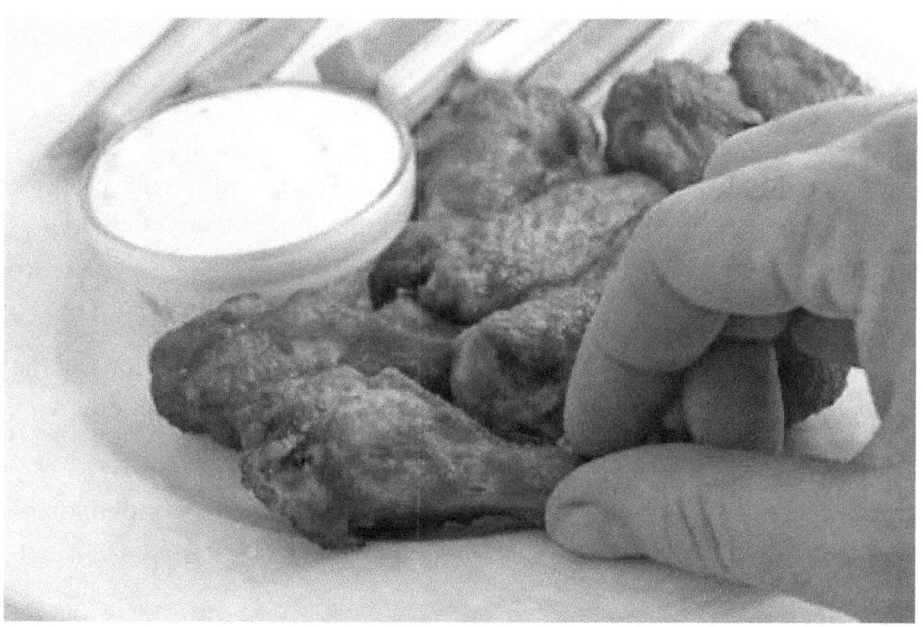

Health Learning Series

M. Usman

Mendon Cottage Books

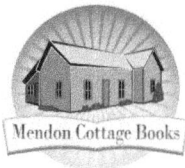

JD-Biz Publishing

Disclaimer

The information is this book is provided for informational purposes only. It is not intended to be used and medical advice or a substitute for proper medical treatment by a qualified health care provider. The information is believed to be accurate as presented based on research by the author.

The contents have not been evaluated by the U.S. Food and Drug Administration or any other Government or Health Organization and the contents in this book are not to be used to treat cure or prevent disease.

The author or publisher is not responsible for the use or safety of any diet, procedure or treatment mentioned in this book. The author or publisher is not responsible for errors or omissions that may exist.

Warning

The Book is for informational purposes only and before taking on any diet, treatment or medical procedure, it is recommended to consult with your primary health care provider.

Our books are available at

1. Amazon.com
2. Barnes and Noble
3. Itunes
4. Kobo
5. Smashwords
6. Google Play Books

Table of Contents

Prelude

What began as a social service has now become a means to earn money and fill one's pockets; specific eating patterns or diets have long been used to get rid of an ailment or condition. The technological boom, along with the ever increasing cleverness of the marketing industry, has resulted in the release of a number of diets that could do "wonders" for you. The wonders part is definitely true, but the kinds of wonders most of them do come at great costs, therefore, it's time to rethink as to where it all went wrong. A simple answer arises: we became modern. That's right, we became modern and abandoned the techniques through which our ancestors survived. Also, we became so disillusioned with our lives that we fell into the simple trap of "making our lives better, the easy way"; that's all you need to think about now.

A simple glimpse of the Paleo Diet is that it's the diet that was followed by our ancestors, well over 10,000 years ago. At that time it was the only diet and comprised of raw foods like meat. Moreover, at that time, humans had to rely on their natural skills for cooking the meal too, as there was rarely a sustainable living atmosphere at that time. This is the basis of the diet that will be used in this book to make your life better in every aspect.

Also it must be known that many practitioners started creating their own personalized versions of the Paleo Diet, however in this book the pure & original version of the Paleo Diet will be used without any additives.

Get ready and flip over.

Getting Started

Chapter 1: Overview

As said before, the Paleo Diet isn't new; it's been around for thousands of years and it definitely isn't something developed in a lab by some professor. The diet is a natural one that created itself after rigorous challenges were placed in front of the primitive man to fill his stomach. There were no grocery stores, super markets, or fast food chains at that time, so man had to search for his food, hunt it down and then find fuel to cook it on. Therefore, don't take the Paleo Diet as just another diet, but a life style that will reinvigorate your living persona.

The Paleo Diet was revived during the 1970s by Gastroenterologist Walter L. Voegtlin. This sparked an increased amount of interest in the diet and soon research papers were being released by health professionals to endorse the perks of the Paleo Diet. By the '90s the Paleo Diet had gained a considerable share of the fitness market and had a great enthusiastic following.

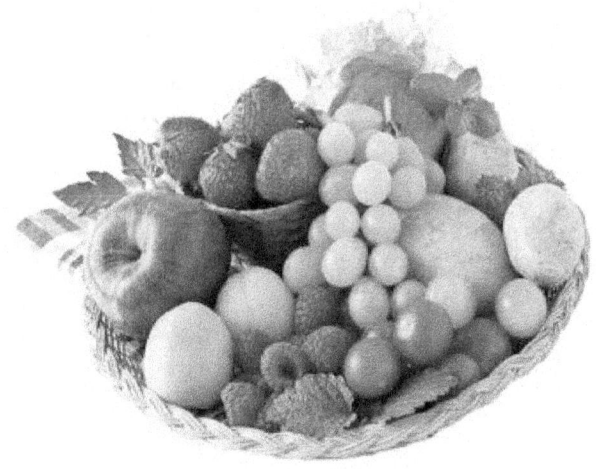

The Paleo Diet, also known as the Caveman Diet, is a combination of all the foods that our ancestors used to consume in the absence of the modern living structure. The concept behind the Paleo Diet is a genetic one; our DNA has not significantly altered, evolved or changed over the past 40 thousand years but our living patterns marginally have. Thus, our bodies have not fully reformed and become compatible to the highly processed and artificial foods that have become an essential part of our lives.

The Paleo Diet consists of anything that can be hunted and/or gathered. Clearly, hunting is not something that needs to be done nowadays since we have a sophisticated system of storage. Still, the diet must consist of natural products which can be a bit hard to find at times. Examples include meat, raw vegetables, fruits, nuts, eggs, shellfish, roots and honey. Furthermore, dairy, potatoes, legumes, grains and oils should be avoided along with salted stuff and products containing gluten.

It can be seen that the Paleo diet is high on whole foods and low on sugar, sodium, and everything else artificial. The elimination of artificial foods automatically leads to a number of health benefits and the inclusion of whole foods leads to the revival of the body's digestive system. Furthermore, balance is brought back to the body and it is set to the right path. There are many benefits of the Paleo Diet like relief from type-2 diabetes, reduction in cardiovascular disease risk and notable weight loss, which is the primary reason this diet is so famous.

It's time you switch to the Paleo diet as a building amount of evidence from all corners, including medical experts, are suggesting that a high protein diet, like the Paleo Diet, can reduce the risk of a variety of diseases and improve one's lifestyle by great lengths. Research papers published by researchers like Dr. Loran Cordain, have categorically stated that Paleolithic diets can prove effective against diseases that affect the cardiovascular system, blood, and lifestyle in general.

Chapter 2: What to Eat and What Not?

Heard of packed foods? Well, there won't be many on a Paleolithic menu. More than 31 percent of Americans consume packaged foods, rather than fresh foods, which lead to problems that in turn result in empty pockets!

Foods that are considered healthy when on the Paleo Diet:

- Lean red meats,

- Organ meats,

- Game meats,

- Poultry,

- Pork,

- Fish & shellfish,

- Eggs,

- Leafy vegetables,

- Mushrooms,

- Root Vegetables,

- Fruits & nuts

Moreover, in small amounts honey, dry fruits, olive oil, coconut oil and animal fats are also allowed.

Foods not recommended while following the Paleo regimen include:

- Grains like corn, barley, oats, rye, rice & wheat,

- Dairy products,

- Beans or legumes,

- Refined salt,

- Refined fats,

- Canned meats,

- Bacon,

- Sodas & packed juices.

These guidelines are quite clear and there's little that's gray. In a nutshell all foods that have been processed, cultivated, or aren't whole need to be out of the kitchen.

Chapter 3: Switching to the Paleo Diet

Some people find switching to the Paleo Diet an extremely difficult task and make it even harder for themselves by keeping the same negative mind set. All that is required to make a smooth shift to the Paleo lifestyle is some good faith, determination, and a little guidance. The process may turn out to be a little uneasy for some, but is not at all painful; think of it as a detox. If you're an athlete then this is the best case and the phase will be less noticeable to you due to the already high consumption of fruits & proteins.

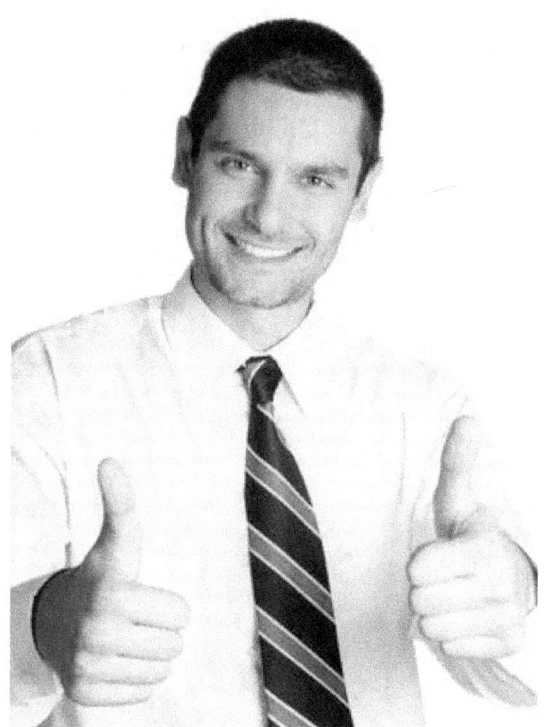

The first rule that must be remembered at all times is: don't go cold turkey. Do everything in a moderate and well chalked out manner. First, get rid of all the processed foods in the house like bread, rice, potato chips, cereal, cakes and pasta. Then start lowering your carbohydrate intake as the week progresses. After one week passes incorporate fresh vegetables into your diet, given that you already consume protein on a daily basis. Start cooking meals in olive oil, corn oil, or other unsaturated fats, avoiding ghee at all costs. Don't drink fizzy drinks and stay limited to water, maple syrup or lemon juice. During the next week remove all packed foods that contain additives like chips, biscuits, and juices from your diet and resort to whole, fresh foods.

After a day or two of going Paleo you might start noticing a few withdrawal symptoms like occasional energy losses. Don't panic, as these will pass and only indicate that your body is shifting to the new diet. Actually, your body starts switching to fat as primary source of energy, thus resulting in the urges of getting something sweet to eat.

But after a week you will start to feel good and content. The soothing feeling of satisfaction will return and you will soon notice minimum untimed energy drops. Your craving for fat & artificial foods will diminish and you'll be set on a path to a better life.

Congratulations as you've just prepared your body for the Paleo Diet.

Chapter 4: Paleo Diet Comparison Chart

The following is a chart that compares the basic features of the Paleo Diet to other popular diets in the market.

	Simple carbohydrates	Saturated fats	Food restrictions	Cost Effective	Health Benefits	A lot of homework	Exercise Compulsory
Paleo	No	Yes	Yes	Yes	Yes	No	No
Weight Watchers	Yes	Yes	No	No	Some	Yes	No
Biggest Loser	Yes	Yes	Some	Some	Yes	Yes	Yes
Jenny Craig	No	Yes	Yes	No	Yes	Yes	Yes
Raw Food	Some	Yes	Yes	No	Some	Yes	No

Benefits of Paleo Diet

Chapter 1: Weight-Loss

The first and foremost benefit of choosing the Paleo Diet is weight loss. It is one of the diet's biggest selling points. It must be known that the body is designed in a way that it must lose the extra calories consumed, but when too many calories are consumed over a long duration of time the body accumulates them which lead to weight gain. When your diet is loaded with carbohydrates and saturated fats, the body's metabolic processes are jammed and the extra calories have to be stored. Many researchers put the initial number of calories per day to be 2500 if one is to start gaining weight. The Paleo diet on the other hand is low in calories and uses proteins & fats as sources of energy, decreasing the strain on the body's metabolic processes.

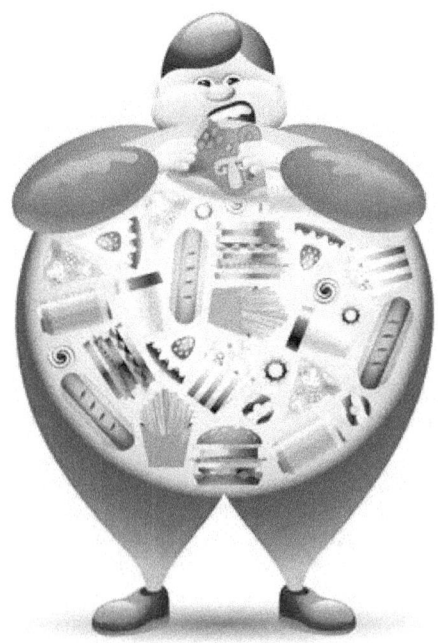

The body works on glucose, which is a form of sugar. This glucose can be prepared in only two ways; either by using carbohydrates or by using other sources. If carbohydrates are present in your body then the liver will go for this and only after this source has been completely exhausted will the whole system get ready for burning fat. Therefore, even if foods containing proteins and fats are consumed along with ample carbohydrates, the body won't benefit from it and you won't lose any weight.

But what happens when a food classified as Paleolithic is consumed? First, the liver stores glucose in the body by converting it into glycogen. Then, when the body has finished digesting any consumed carbohydrates, the liver starts to convert this glycogen back into glucose. As the carbohydrates are not in abundance in the Paleo diet, the glycogen reserves run out and the body has to resort to other sources like fat. The body breaks down fat cells and the liver manufactures chemicals from these cells that are then used as fuel. This is how the body loses weight when on the Paleo diet.

To further understand as to how the body loses weight, you must understand that in order to produce burnable fuel the body must render the properties of insulin. Insulin is the real culprit in this entire scenario, as insulin raises the glucose levels.

- Producing glucose by breaking down proteins,

- Decreasing the breakdown of glucose,

Also, it keeps the body from burning fat which results in more fat being stored in the body than being burnt. But, the Paleo Diet tackles this problem by eliminating carbohydrates from the diet. When carbohydrates are eliminated, that means sugar is no longer the primary source of fuel for the body.

Chapter 2: Reduces Type-2 Diabetes Risk

The Paleo Diet is not only good at keeping extra weight off of you, but also can deal with the increasing problem of type-2 diabetes. Increased popularity of the diet resulted in a wide array of research being launched on the diet. One particular area showed that the diet can help diabetics manage their blood sugar.

In 2011, a study was launched at the UCSF that found that type-2 diabetics who followed the Paleo Diet showed great improvements in blood sugar levels, blood pressure, and cholesterol by significant amounts. At the same time, participants who were kept on the traditional diet of the American Diabetics Association showed little improvement. It is to be noted that enough food was provided to each participant so that the benefits didn't come from loss of weight.

At the moment, scientists aren't sure as to how the Paleo Diet works, but some researchers are coming to the conclusion that all carbohydrates aren't equal. Carbohydrates obtained from fruits & vegetables are much better than those from grains. Furthermore, fruits and vegetables contain antioxidants that further enhance the beneficial effect of these carbohydrates.

One particular study, known as the Jonsson study, was the first to analyze the potential benefit of the Paleo Diet on patients of type-2 diabetes. The study contained 13 subjects, all type-2 diabetics and on oral therapy. The study went on for 3 months, during which the subjects were given either a Paleolithic diet followed by a diabetic diet or the diets in the opposite order. Compared to the diabetic diet, the Paleo diet left lighter footprints with respect to weight, body mass index, blood pressure and other chemical levels. Conclusively it was found that the Paleo Diet was more superior in terms of relieving the symptoms of type 2 diabetics.

Chapter 3: Builds Muscles

Muscle proteins are made up of BCAAs or branched chain amino acids. These amino acids must come from an external source as they cannot be manufactured inside the body. The only way to acquire them is by eating foods rich in this amino acid like lean meat, chicken, beef and turkey. The Paleo Diet fundamentally consists of these food items; therefore, consuming BCAAs are no problem for a person on the diet.

The Paleo Diet can prove quite beneficial, especially for athletes, as they are always looking to gain more muscle than fat. During physical workouts, they need a huge amount of energy as their metabolism becomes extremely fast paced. First, the existing carbohydrate reserves are depleted and after that BCAAs are used as fuel. Thus, it is only logical that a diet rich in BCAAs be consumed in order to prevent breakdown of extra muscles. When the body is under stress it starts to break down proteins. In contrast, BCAAs aid in the release of a hormone, called testosterone, which aids muscle growth. The gain in mass of your body will be dependent upon the ratio of the two chemicals thus, the greater the amount of BCAAs the more you will gain muscle.

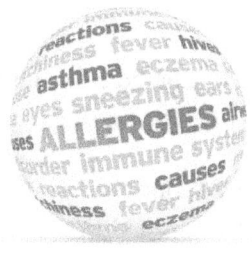

Chapter 4: Other Benefits

The Paleo Diet sets your whole body on a path of better health. The following are the general benefits of consuming the Paleo Diet:

- The elimination of artificial foods from one's diet results in the successive elimination of harmful additives, flavorings and compounds that are toxic to health.

- Paleo diet is not all about proteins; it contains a healthy amount of fruits, vegetables and nuts which are all essential for proper nutrient absorption and gut health.

- The Paleo Diet is also low in sodium which helps decrease the feelings of bloating, a common occurrence after eating a western diet. This, combined with a lot of fiber from whole foods, results in a healthy digestive system.

- The energy provided by fats and proteins may prove a little nauseating at first, but later on they will give you a feeling of serenity unlike any other food. The energy provided by proteins is transferred gradually as well as evenly to the body, helping blood sugar remain under control.

- The Paleo Diet provides the body with Omega 3 fatty acids in an amount good for the arteries, skin and brain to function.

- The Paleo Diet also helps in improving cognitive functions like sleeping patterns, improvement in mood, and mental clarity making it an all-round package for any individual.

Breakfast Recipes

Chapter 1: Paleo Bread

Makes: 6 servings

Prep time: 15 minutes

Cooking time: 15 minutes

Ingredients:

- 2 large plantains, peeled and broken
- 2 eggs
- 1 tablespoon olive oil
- Salt

Directions:

Preheat an oven to 350 degrees Fahrenheit and line a baking sheet with parchment paper. Blend the plantain, eggs, olive oil, and salt to taste in a food processor until a smooth mixture is obtained. Spread the mixture into a rectangle, ½ inch thick, onto the baking sheet, sprinkling some more salt on the top. Bake this in the oven until the bread is light brown in color which will take about 15 minutes. Give the bread 5 minutes to cool before slicing it.

Chapter # 2: Paleo Pancakes

Makes: 10 servings

Prep time: 10 minutes

Cooking time: 20 minutes

Ingredients:

- 2 eggs

- 1 ½ cup almond meal

- ½ teaspoon vanilla extract

- ½ cup applesauce

- ½ teaspoon cinnamon

- ¼ teaspoon baking powder

- ¼ cup coconut milk

- 1 teaspoon olive oil

- 1 cup strawberries

Directions:

Mix together the eggs, almond flour, cinnamon, vanilla, baking powder, applesauce, and coconut milk in a big bowl. Take an oiled griddle and place over medium heat. Drop the batter by large spoonfuls on it and cook until bubbles appear and the edges of pancake are dry. Flip and cook until the other side is browned as well. Repeat this with the remaining batter. Puree the strawberries in a food processor and top the pancakes with them.

Chapter # 3: Zucchini & Eggs

Makes: 1 serving

Prep time: 5 minutes

Cooking time: 5 minutes

Ingredients:

- 1 egg

- 2 teaspoons olive oil

- 1 small zucchini

- Salt & pepper

Directions:

Heat a skillet over medium heat. Pour a little oil onto it, sautéing the zucchini until it turns tender. Spread the zucchini in a layered form and pour some beaten eggs on top of it. Cook until the egg becomes firm and then season with salt & pepper.

Main Dishes

Chapter # 1: Paleo Chili

Makes: 4 servings

Prep time: 15 minutes

Cooking time: 35 minutes

Ingredients:

- 1 tablespoon chili powder
- 1 dried chipotle pepper
- 1 tablespoon ground cumin
- 1 teaspoon oregano
- 1 cup boiling water
- 1 ½ teaspoon coconut oil
- 1 teaspoon unsweetened cocoa
- 1 cup yellow onion, chopped
- 1 teaspoon Worcestershire sauce
- 1 cup green bell pepper, chopped
- 1 cup red bell pepper, chopped
- 1 can crushed tomatoes
- 4 garlic cloves

- 1 ½ teaspoon kosher salt

- 1 pound bison

- ½ teaspoon black pepper

- ½ pound ground pork sausage

Directions:

Soak the chipotle pepper in boiling water so that it softens, which will be about 10 minutes. Remove the pepper from the water and mince it. Melt the coconut oil over medium heat. Cook the onion, red bell pepper and green bell pepper until it is tender, which will take 10 minutes maximum. Stir the garlic and minced chipotle into the onion mixture and cook until it turns fragrant. Stir in the bison and sausage in the onion mixture and cook until the meat is brown and crumbly; this will take another 10 minutes. Stir in the cumin, oregano, chili powder, Worcestershire sauce, and cocoa powder into the bison mixture followed by tomatoes and salt. Bring it to a boil and reduce the heat to low, simmering until the flavors settle down.

Chapter # 2: Baked Salmon

Makes: 2 servings

Prep time: 15 minutes

Cooking time: 45 minutes

Ingredients:

- 2 cloves garlic
- 1 teaspoon black pepper
- 6 tablespoons olive oil
- 1 tablespoon lemon juice
- 1 teaspoon dried basil
- 1 tablespoon fresh parsley
- 2 fillets salmon
- 1 teaspoon salt

Directions:

In a medium sized bowl, prepare the marinade by mixing the garlic, basil, olive oil, pepper, salt, lemon juice, and parsley. Then, place the salmon fillets in a medium baking dish and cover it with the marinade. Marinate in the fridge for an hour, turning it occasionally. Preheat an oven to 190 degrees Celsius and place the fillets in aluminum foil, covering them with the marinade and sealing them. Place the sealed salmon in the glass dish and bake for 45 minutes.

Chapter # 3: Rapid Roast Chicken

Makes: 8 servings

Prep time: 15 minutes

Cooking time: 1 hour

Ingredients:

- 1 whole chicken
- ¼ teaspoon dried oregano
- ¼ teaspoon dried basil
- 1 tablespoon olive oil
- ¼ teaspoon salt
- ¼ teaspoon paprika
- ¼ teaspoon ground black pepper
- 1/8 teaspoon cayenne pepper

Directions:

Preheat an oven to 230 degrees Celsius. Rinse the chicken from inside and out under running water and remove every portion of fat; pat dry with towels. Put the chicken in a baking pan, rub it with olive oil, and mix the salt, oregano, pepper, basil and cayenne pepper together and sprinkle it over chicken. Roast the chicken in the preheated oven for about 20 minutes before lowering the heat to 205 degrees Celsius; continue to roast to a minimum internal temperature of 74 degrees Celsius for about 40 more minutes. Let it cool for some time and serve.

Chapter # 4: Paleo Chorizo & Kale Stew

Makes: 8 servings

Prep time: 40 minutes

Cooking time: 45 minutes

Ingredients:

- 1 large onion, diced

- 2 tablespoon olive oil

- 1 pinch saffron threads

- 5 garlic cloves

- 8 ounces Spanish chorizo, cut

- 2 sweet potatoes

- 3 stalks celery

- 8 cups chicken broth

- 3 carrots, diced

- 4 cups dinosaur kale

- 2 teaspoon ground cumin

- 1 lemon

- 1 tablespoon paprika

- ½ teaspoon ground turmeric

- 2 teaspoons kosher salt

- 1 pinch harissa

- 1 teaspoon black pepper

- Salt & pepper

- 1 tablespoon fresh parsley

Directions:

Cook the onion in olive oil over medium-high heat for 5 minutes. Add the chorizo and cook along with stirring for another 3 minutes. Add the carrots and celery and continue to stir until the vegetables have softened; this will take about 3 minutes. Add paprika, cumin, turmeric, black pepper, kosher salt, garlic, and saffron threads. Cook until the garlic is soft. Add the sweet potatoes plus the chicken broth and bring the pot to a boil and reduce the heat to low, still cooking until the potatoes are tender. Add the kale and cook until the vegetables become significantly soft and the kale is wilted through. Stir in the lemon juice, salt and some pepper; garnish with harissa and parsley and serve.

Chapter # 5: Spaghetti Squash with Sauce

Makes: 8 servings

Prep time: 40 minutes

Cooking time: 30 minutes

Ingredients:

- ¼ cup water
- 1 red bell pepper
- 1 spaghetti squash
- 1 14.5 ounce can crushed tomatoes
- 1 ½ pounds ground beef
- 1 8 ounce can crushed tomatoes
- 1 diced white onion
- ¼ cup chopped fresh basil
- 1 tablespoon virgin olive oil
- ¼ cup chopped oregano
- 1 cup sliced mushrooms
- ¼ cups chopped thyme
- 1 zucchini
- 1 tablespoon red pepper flakes

- 1 green bell pepper

- ½ cup virgin olive oil

Directions:

Preheat an oven to 200 degrees Celsius. Pour some water in a baking dish and place halves of the squash into it; roast them until they turn tender, which will be almost 40 minutes. While the squash is roasting, cook and stir the beef and onions in a skillet over medium heat until the beef is crumbly and evenly browned. Drain and discard the extra grease and set the beef aside. Heat a tablespoon of olive oil in a skillet over medium heat. Cook the mushrooms, green bell peppers, red bell peppers, and zucchini, both of the crushed tomatoes, oregano, basil and thyme. Simmer this over medium heat until the vegetables are tender. Add the ground beef and onions, stir them in and simmer on low heat while the spaghetti squash is finished. Scrape the spaghetti squash halves with a fork and shred the squash to strands. Drizzle each serving of squash with a tablespoon of virgin olive oil and top each one with a chunk of meat sauce.

Chapter # 6: Homemade Pastrami

Makes: 1, 4 pound pastrami

Prep time: 1 hour 35 minutes

Cooking time: 6 hours 10 minutes

Ingredients:

- 2 cloves crushed garlic
- 1 teaspoon dry mustard
- ½ cup vegetable oil
- ¼ cup ground black pepper
- ½ teaspoon white pepper
- ¼ teaspoon cayenne pepper
- 2 tablespoons paprika
- 4 pounds corned beef
- 2 teaspoons ground coriander

Directions:

Mix the garlic and vegetable oil in a bowl and set them aside for an hour.

Next, preheat an oven to 110 degrees Celsius. Combine the paprika, coriander, black pepper, dry mustard, cayenne pepper, and white pepper in a large bowl. Set them aside. Take a sheet of aluminum foil and cover a baking sheet with it. Coat the aluminum foil with the garlic-oil and lay the corned beef brisket on the foil. Brush the remaining garlic-oil and pepper mixture onto the corned beef, saving just 2 teaspoons of the pepper mixture. Making sure that the fat side of the beef is facing up and wrap it in aluminum sheets, placing the wrapped beef on another sheet with the fat side down. Place this beef on a third sheet of aluminum and wrap again. Bake for 6 hours; remove the pastrami from the oven and let it cool. With the pastrami still wrapped, place it in a plastic bag and refrigerate it for 8 hours. Preheat the broiler and set the oven rack at about 6 inches from the source. Line a baking sheet with aluminum foil, remove pastrami form the refrigerator, unwrap and place it on the baking sheet. Sprinkle it with the saved pepper mixture and place it in the oven. Broil briefly until the surface becomes brown. Remove the pastrami from the oven and cut slices about 1/8 inches thick.

Heat a skillet over low heat and place the slices on the skillet; pour a few drops of water. Heat it for about 5 minutes, or until the fat changes color from white to translucent.

Others

Chapter # 1: Parrothead Salad

Makes: 6 servings

Prep time: 20 minutes

Cooking time: 10 minutes

Ingredients:

- 1 head leaf lettuce

- ½ cup raisins

- ½ pound fresh strawberries

- ¼ cup toasted slivered almonds

- ½ pound fresh blueberries

- ¼ cup chopped red onion

- 4 slices bacon

- 1 mango seeded & peeled

- 1 cup cherry tomatoes

Directions:

Toss the strawberries, lettuce, blueberries, mango, tomatoes, almonds, raisins, and onions in a bowl. Cover it and refrigerate for 30 minutes so that all flavors can settle in. Place the bacon in a large skillet and cook over medium heat, with occasional turns, until it becomes crisp; this will take only 10 minutes. Drain the bacon slices, crumble them & sprinkle over the salad and serve.

Chapter # 2: Banana Bread

Makes: 12 slices

Prep time: 15 minutes

Cooking time: 45 minutes

Ingredients:

- ½ cup water

- 1 serving cooking spray

- 2 cups almond flour

- 1 teaspoon almond extract

- 1 tablespoon cinnamon

- ¼ cup agave syrup

- 1 teaspoon baking soda

- 2 ripe bananas

- 2 eggs

Directions:

Preheat an oven to 175 degrees Celsius and spray cooking spray over a loaf pan. Mix together the baking soda, cinnamon, and almond flour in a bowl. Beat two eggs into another bowl and add water, agave syrup, almond extract and mashed bananas to this. Add this mixture into the flour mixture, mixing until no dry area is visible. Pour the batter onto the loaf pan. Bake the bread in the oven until it turns brown and crisp; this will take 45 minutes.

Chapter # 3: Coconut-Dark Chocolate Chip Cookies

Makes: 24 cookies

Prep time: 20 minutes

Cooking time: 10 minutes

Ingredients:

- ¼ cup honey

- 2 cups almond flour

- 1 ½ teaspoons coconut oil

- 2/3 cups unsweetened coconut

- 1 teaspoon vanilla extract

- 1/3 cup coconut flour

- ¾ cups dark chocolate chips

- 1 egg

- ½ cup almond butter

Directions:

Preheat an oven to 175 degrees Celsius. Mix the shredded coconut, almond flour, and coconut flour together. Beat the egg in a large bowl and mix in the honey, almond butter, vanilla extract, and coconut oil into the egg. Stir in the chocolate chips into the dough and mix until they are combined. Scoop the dough into small balls and place them 1 inch apart on an ungreased baking sheet; bake for 10 minutes.

Chapter # 4: Grapefruit & Avocado Salad

Makes: 4 servings

Prep time: 15 minutes

Cooking time: 15 minutes

Ingredients:

- 3 tablespoons olive oil
- 2 pink grapefruits, sectioned
- 1 large avocado, diced
- 1 cup alfalfa sprouts
- 1 lemon
- 1 pinch salt
- 1 pinch black pepper

Directions:

Arrange a quarter of the grapefruit and a quarter of avocado onto a salad plate; top them up with a quarter of the sprouts. Repeat these steps until you make 4 salads. Mix the lemon juice, olive oil, salt & pepper in bowl and sprinkle over the salad.

Conclusion

The Paleo Diet is all about going back to where we came from. Of course we can't literally do this, but we can imitate it to the level from which we can gain a lot for our bodies. The Paleo Diet has enormous benefits which range from weigh loss to cardiovascular health.

All in all it is a complete package that will drastically change your body's internal workings to bring back its healthy state. All necessary information about the diet has been given in this book so that you face no difficulty or lack of motivation while following the diet.

Whether to change yourself or not? Only you can answer this question.

Best of Luck and stay healthy!

References

http://www.fotolia.com/id/11347590

http://www.fotolia.com/id/42730841

http://www.fotolia.com/id/52133132

http://www.fotolia.com/id/51102457

http://www.fotolia.com/id/42606253

http://www.fotolia.com/id/ 45257208

Author Bio

Muhammad Usman is a distinguished medical graduate of Allama Iqbal medical college (AIMC). He is a professional writer who has been in the field for more than 4 years. During this time he has produced 10,000+ articles, blogs and eBooks on various niches related to diseases, health, fitness, nutrition and well-being. He is a regular contributor to several journals related to medicine and surgery. He is the editor of several journals and newspapers.

Check out some of the other JD-Biz Publishing books

Gardening Series on Amazon

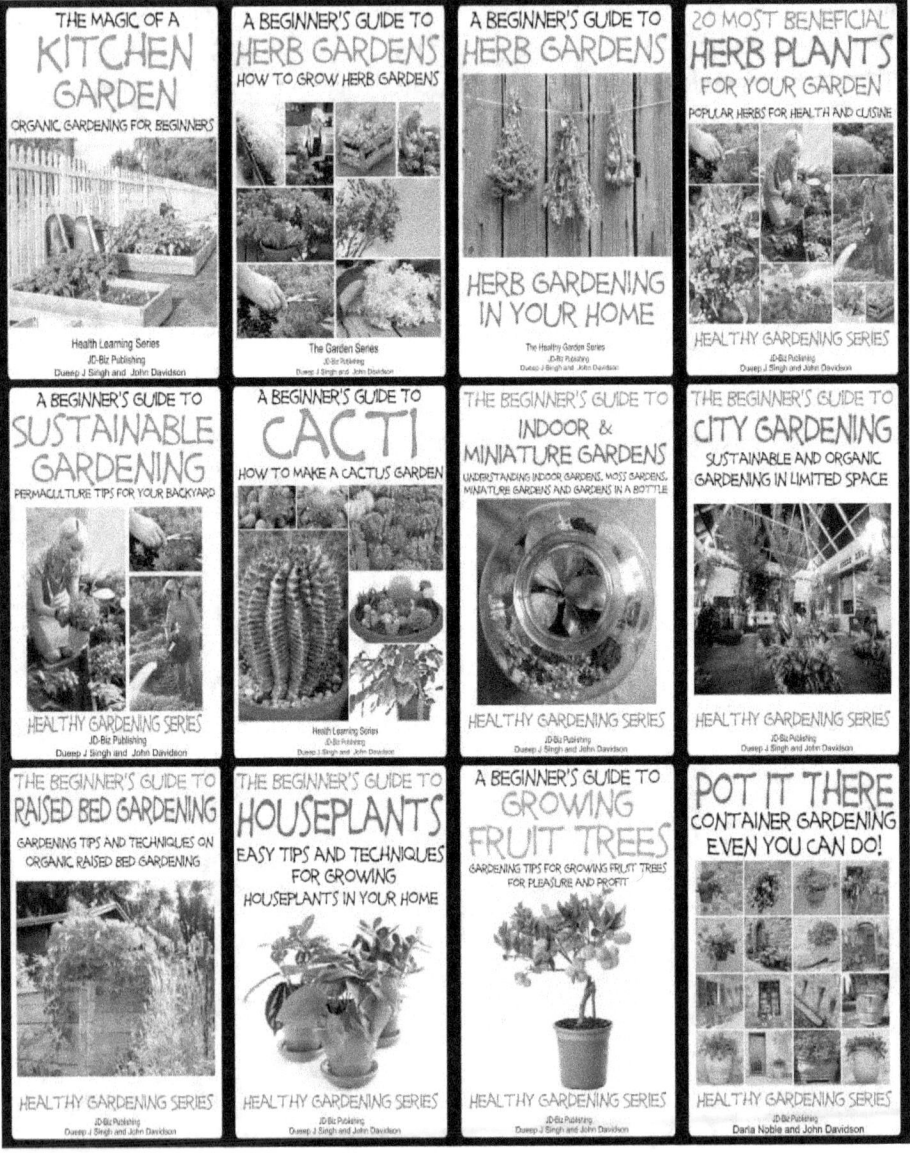

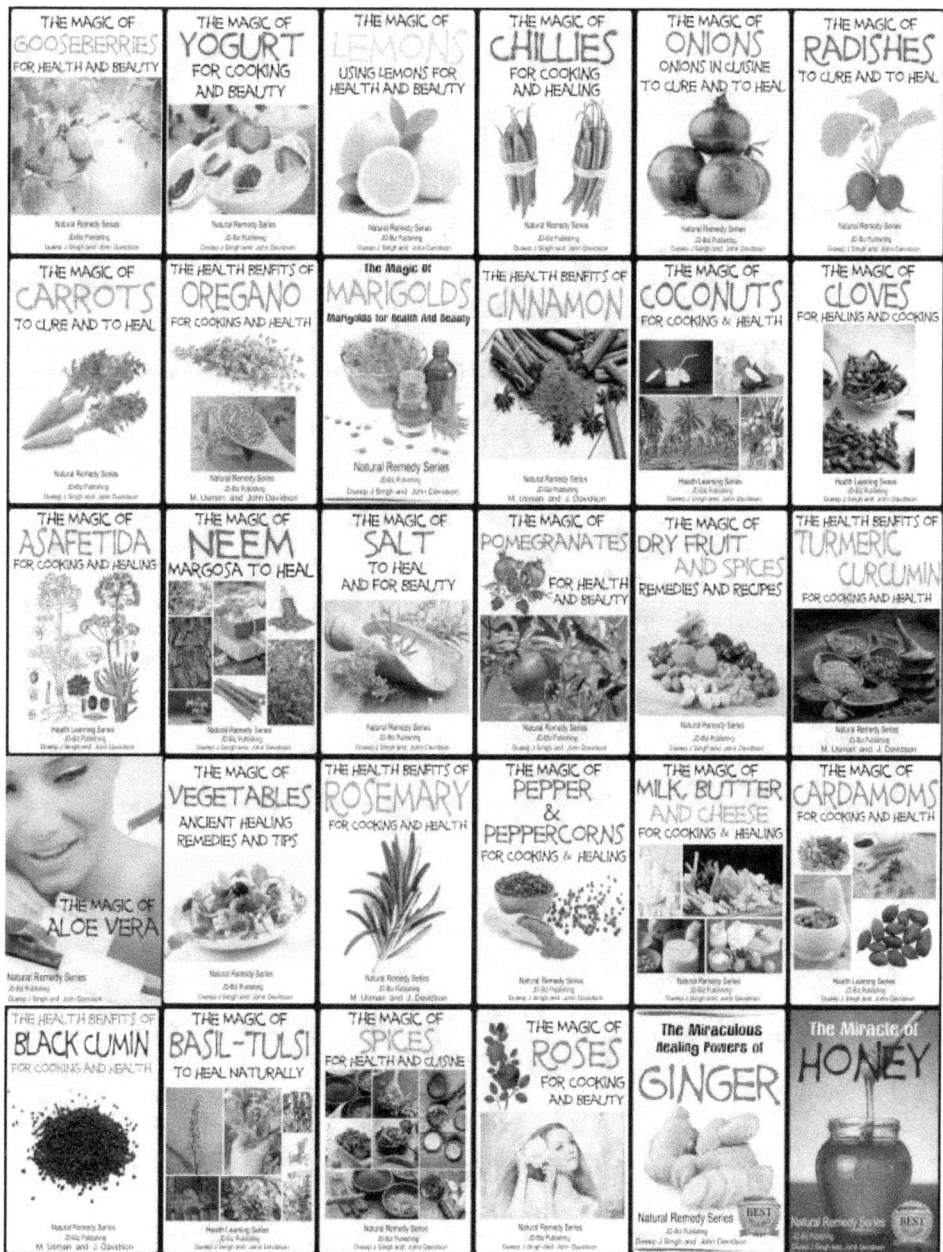

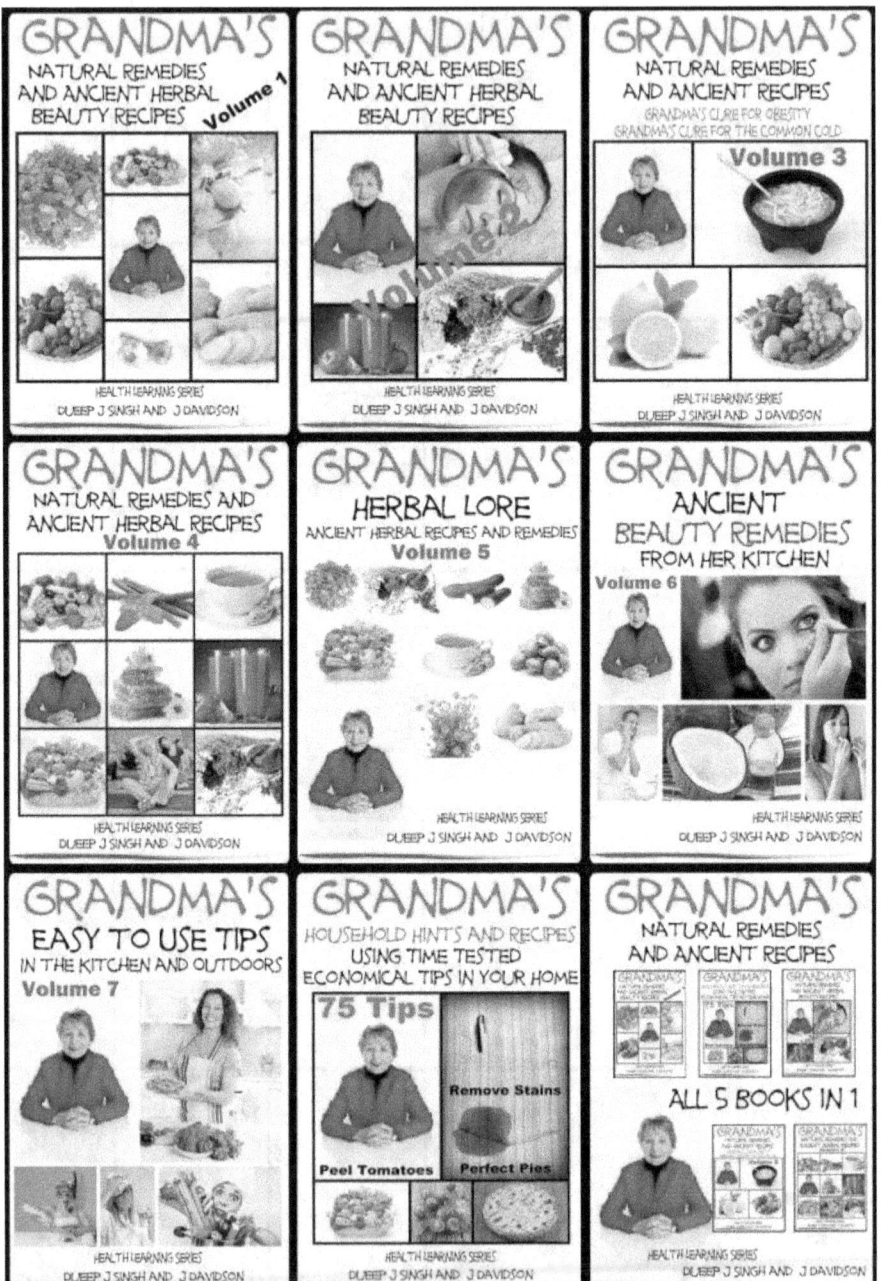

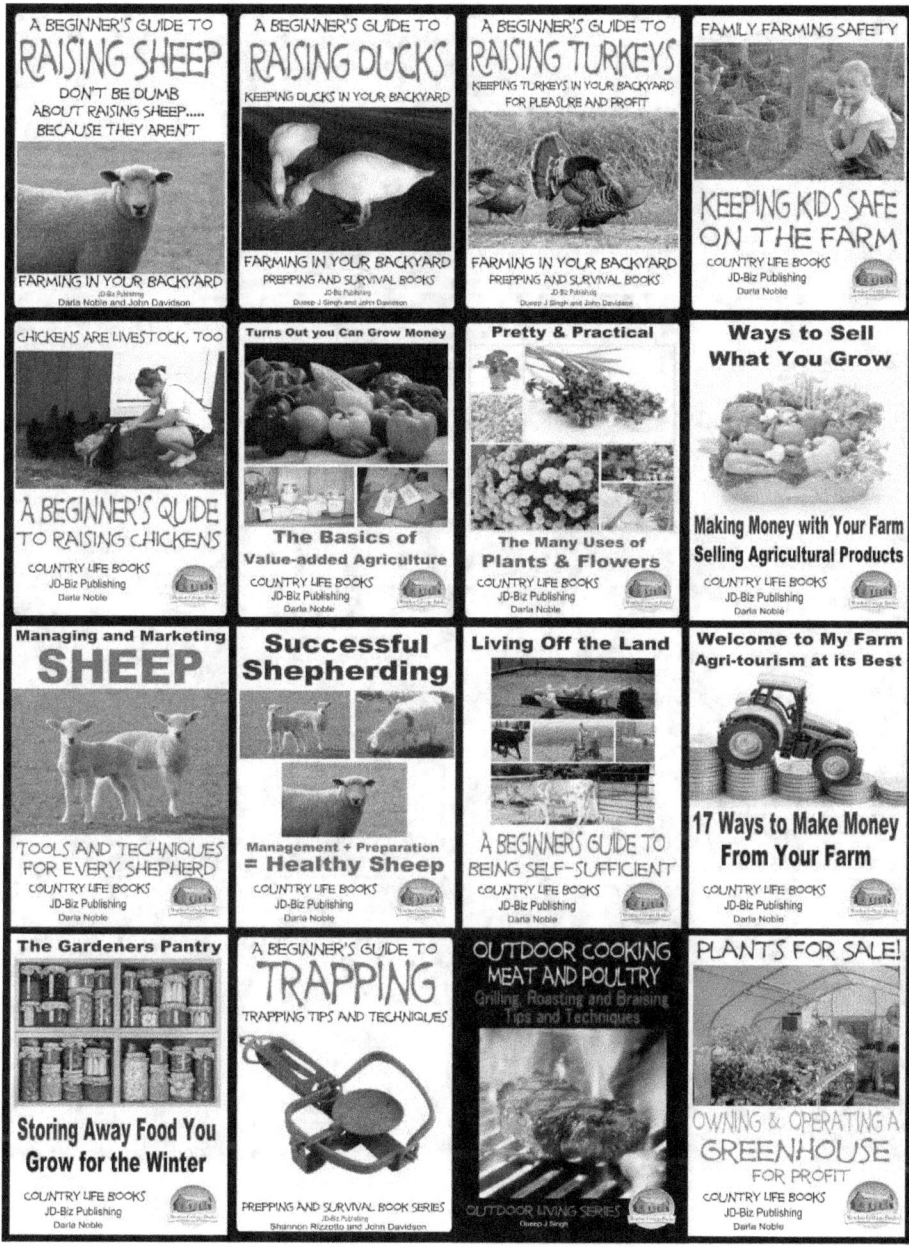

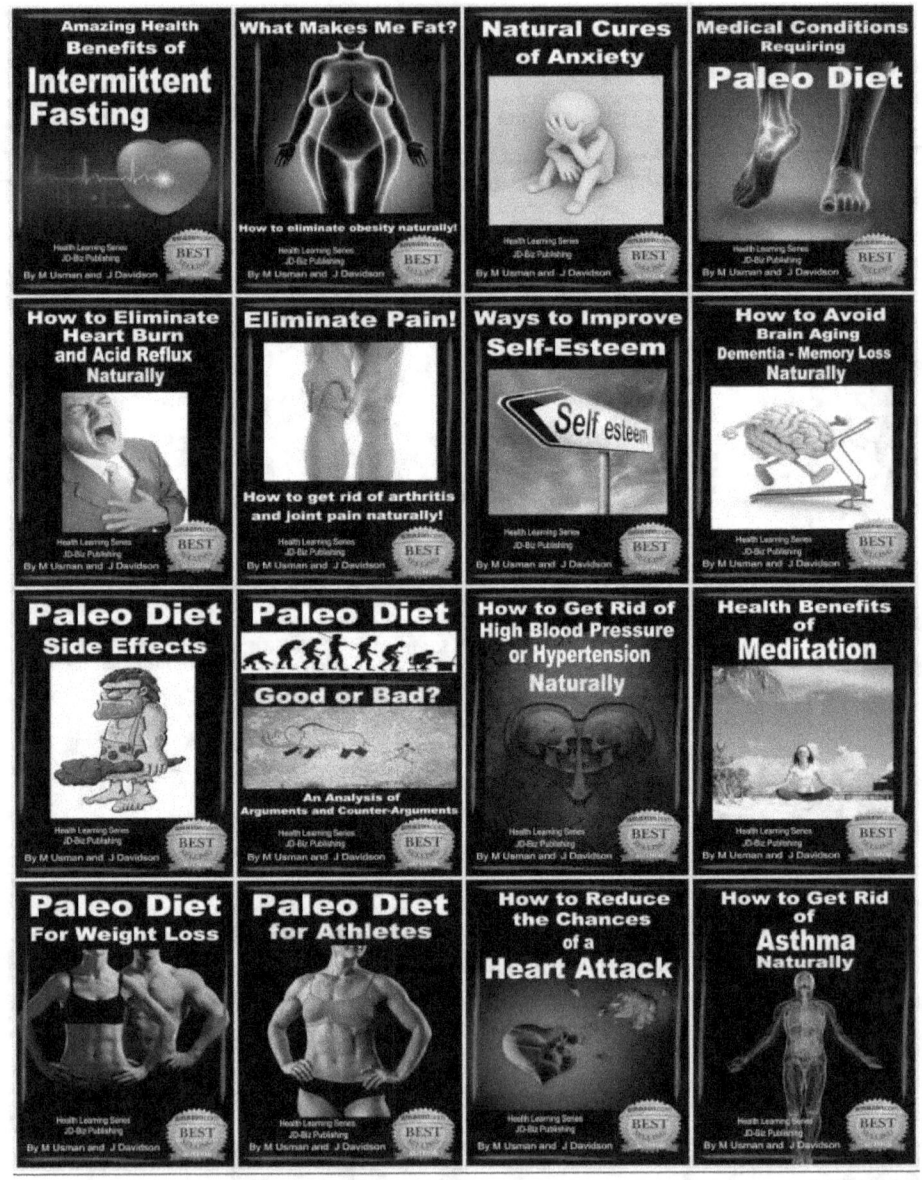

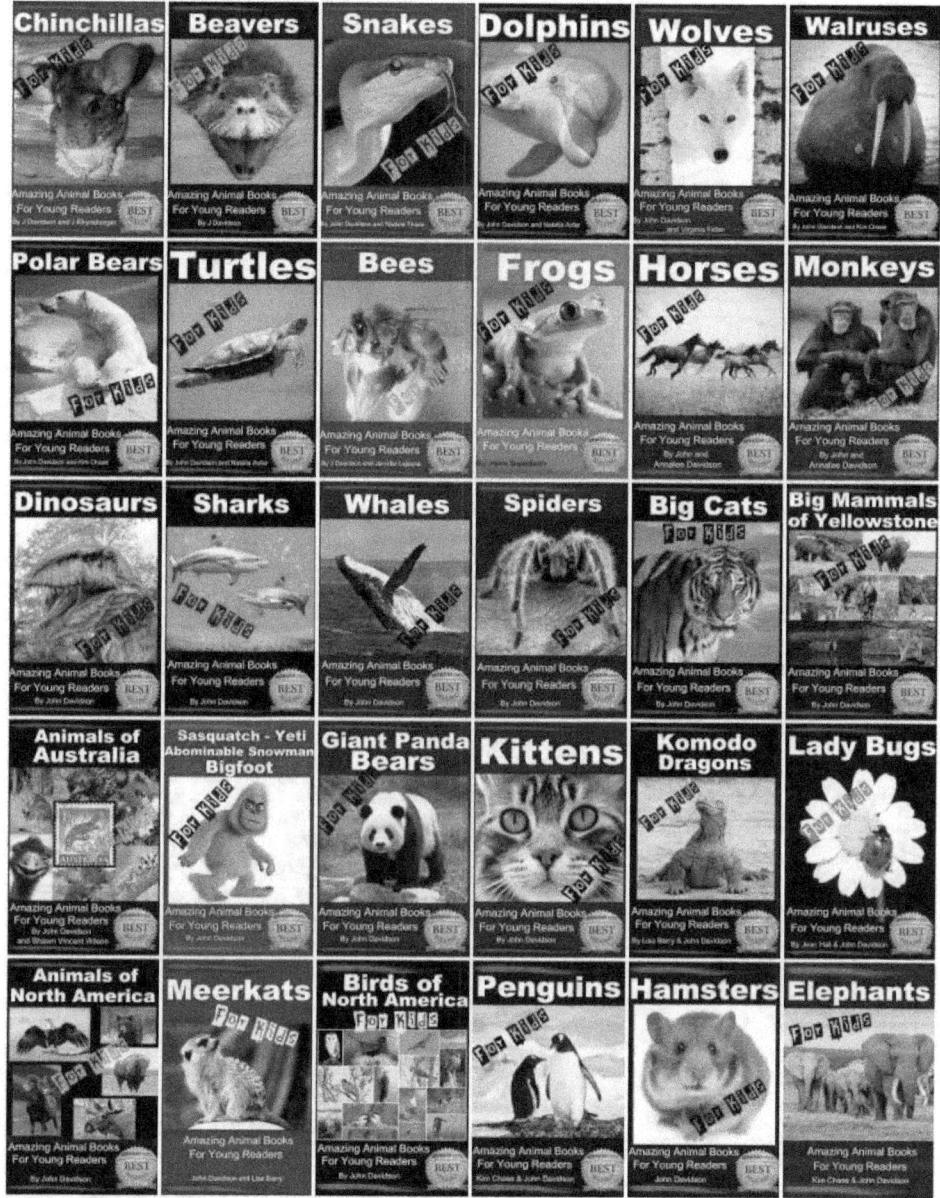

Learn To Draw Series

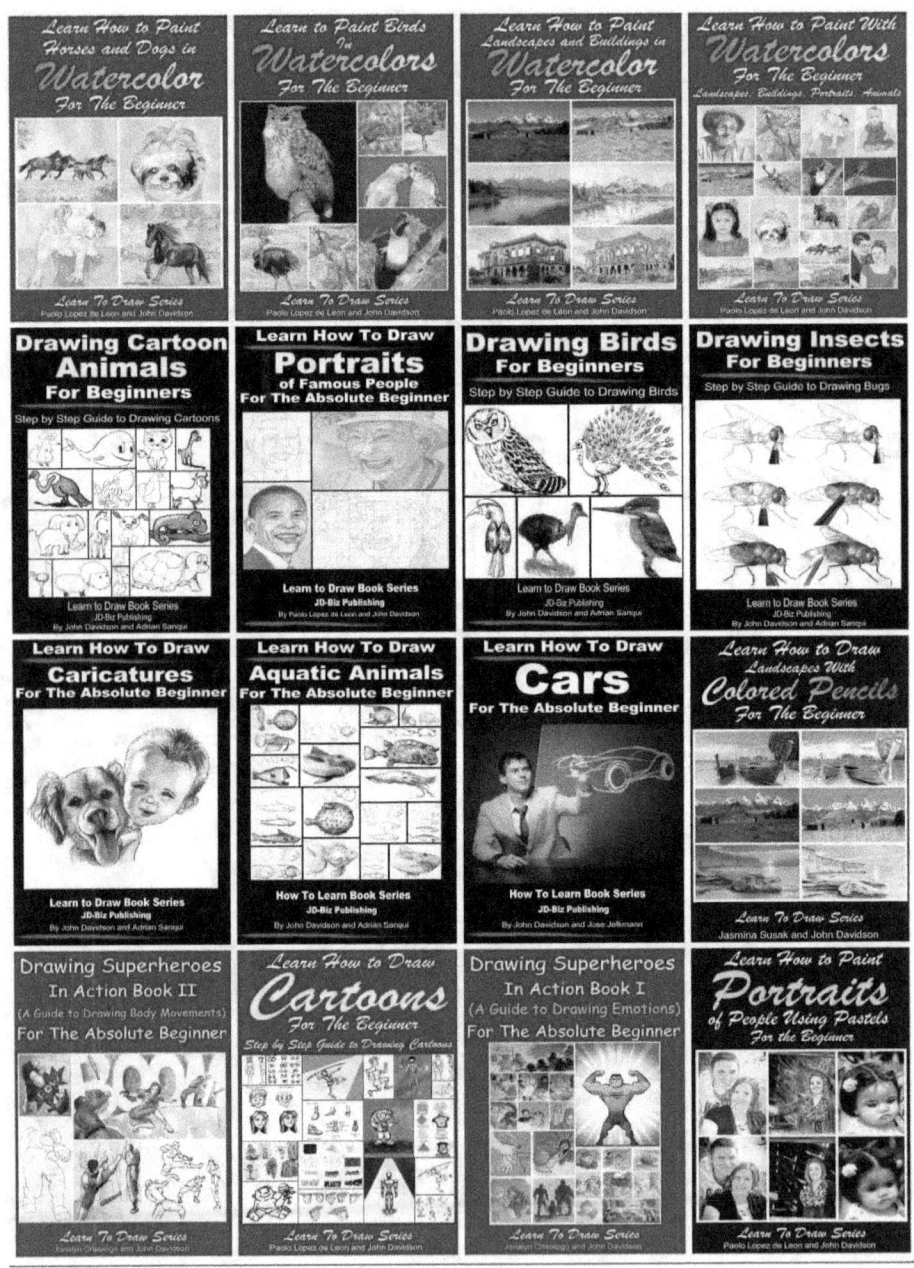

How to Build and Plan Books

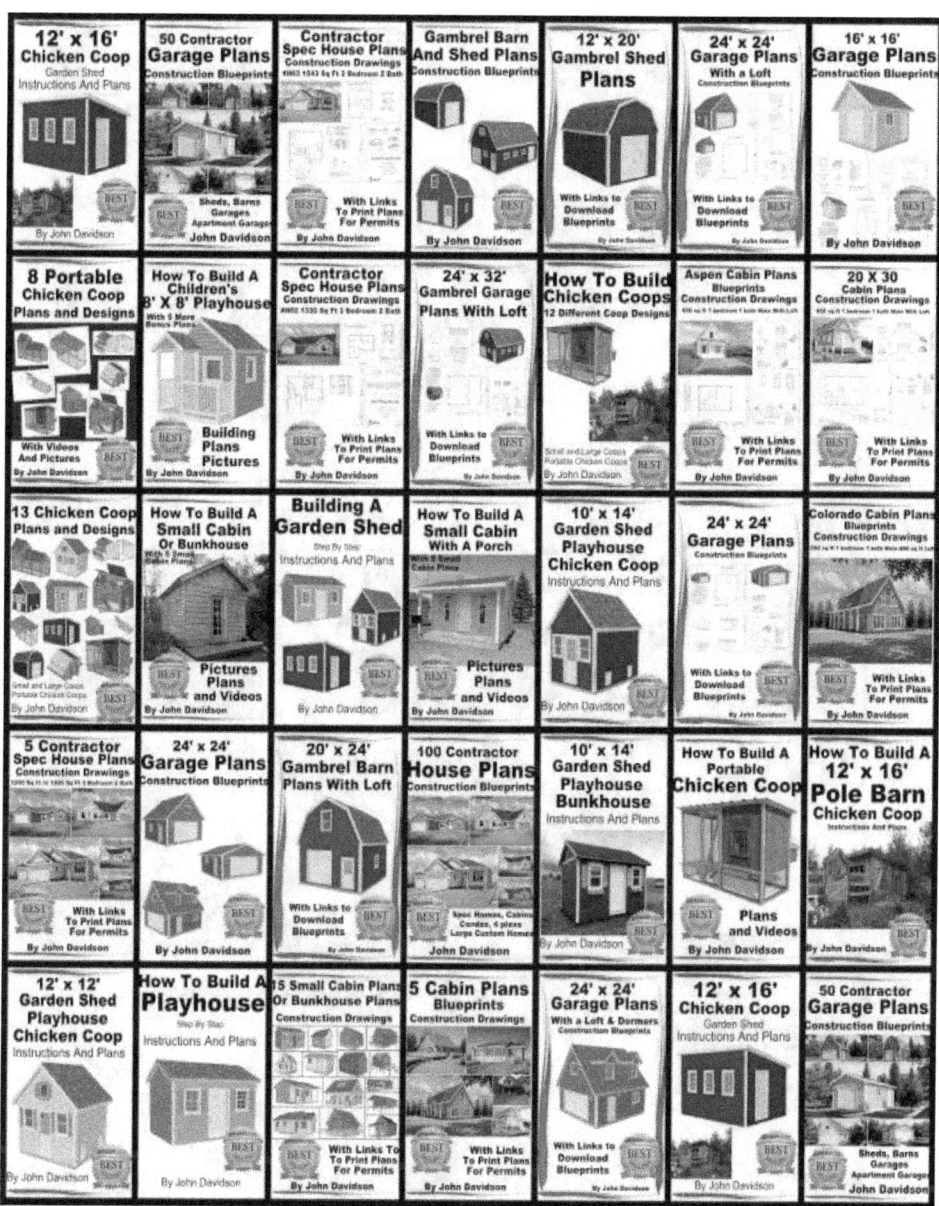

Entrepreneur Book Series

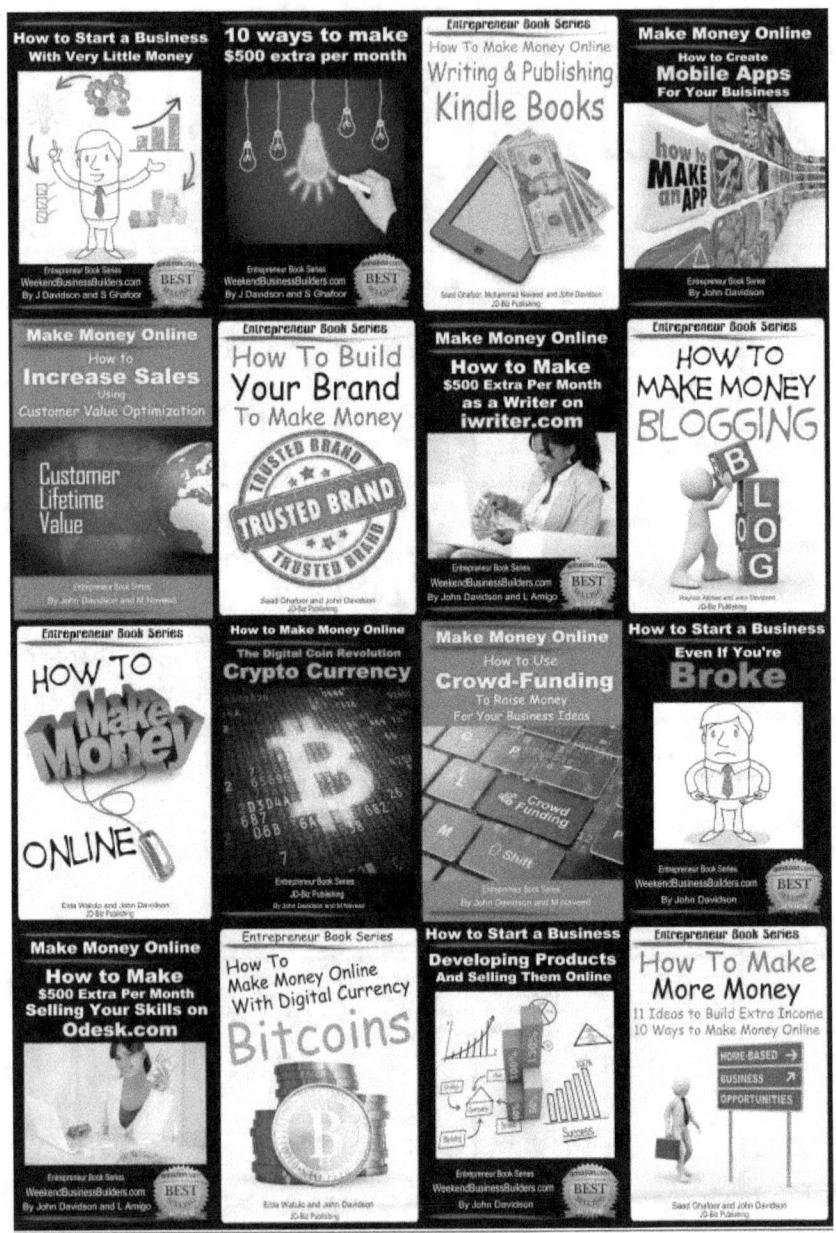

Our books are available at

1. Amazon.com

2. Barnes and Noble

3. Itunes

4. Kobo

5. Smashwords

6. Google Play Books

Publisher

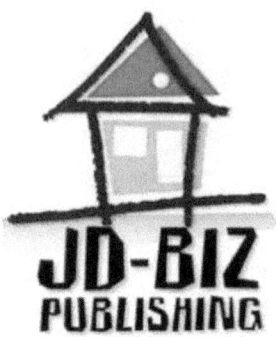

JD-Biz Corp

P O Box 374

Mendon, Utah 84325

http://www.jd-biz.com/

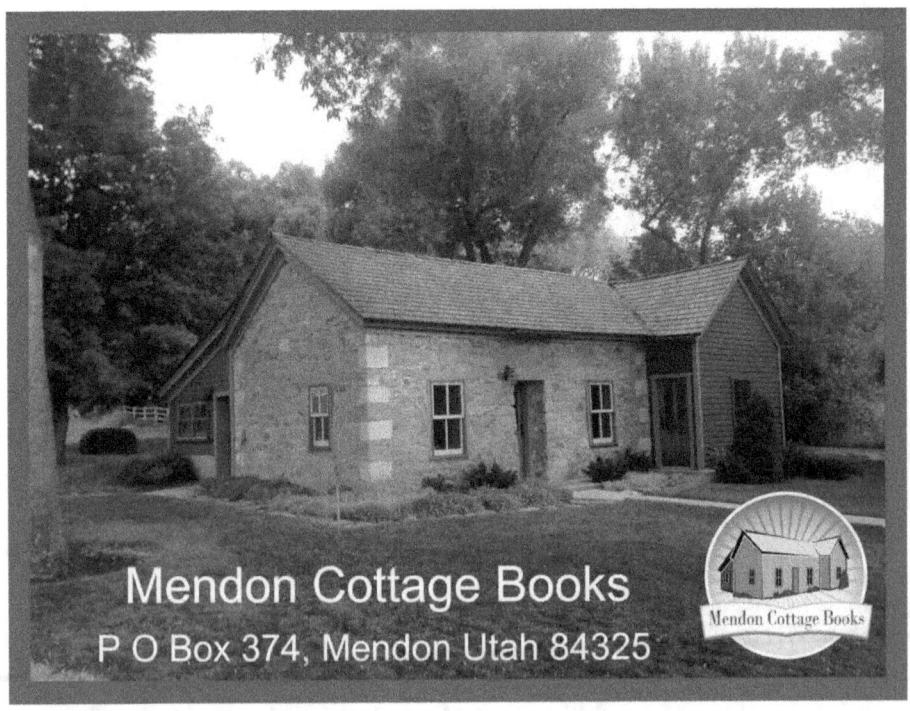